The Healthy
Air Fryer Cookbook

Delicious Dinner Recipes for Cooking Easier, Faster,
for You and Your Family!

Carol Scott

TABLE OF CONTENT

INTRODUCTION

An investment in your health is the best present that you could ever make for yourself. By using the wonderful air-fryer appliance you can prepare healthy foods that taste great while you are in control of what you are eating. You can enjoy that great crunchy taste that will taste like deep-fried foods but when prepared with your air-fryer will be without the extra fat!

This guide has the most delicious-sounding recipes, head to the grocery store and get cooking! That's the only way you can expand your cooking repertoire, improve your skills with your air fryer, learn how to cook mouth-watering and healthy foods and save a ton of time.

It is important to note that air fried foods are still fried. Unless you've decided to eliminate the use of oils in cooking, you must still be cautious about the food you eat. Despite that, it clearly presents a better and healthier option than deep frying. It helps you avoid unnecessary fats and oils, which makes it an ideal companion when you intend to lose weight. It offers a lot more benefits, which include the following:

- It is convenient and easy to use, plus, it's easy to clean.
- It doesn't give off unwanted smells when cooking.
- You can use it to prepare a variety of meals.
- It can withstand heavy cooking.
- It is durable and made of metal and high-grade plastic.

What's the difference between an air fryer and deep fryer? Air fryers bake food at a high temperature with a high-powered fan, while deep fryers cook food in a vat of oil that has been heated up to a specific temperature. Both cook food quickly, but an air fryer requires practically zero preheat time while a deep fryer can take upwards of 10 minutes. Air fryers also require little to no oil and deep fryers require a lot that absorb into the food. Food comes out crispy and juicy in both appliances, but don't taste the same, usually because deep fried foods are coated in batter that cook differently in an air fryer vs a deep fryer. Battered foods needs to be sprayed with oil before cooking in an air fryer to help them color and get crispy, while the hot oil soaks into the batter in a deep fryer. Flour-based batters and wet batters don't cook well in an air fryer, but they come out very well in a deep fryer.

The ketogenic diet is one such example. The diet calls for a very small number of carbs to be eaten. This means food such as rice, pasta, and other starchy vegetables like potatoes are off the menu. Even relaxed versions of the keto diet minimize carbs to a large extent and this compromises the goals of many dieters. They end up having to exert large amounts of willpower to follow the diet. This doesn't do them any favors since willpower is like a muscle. At some point, it tires and this is when the dieter goes right back to their old pattern of eating. I have personal experience with this. In terms of health benefits, the keto diet offers the most. The reduction of carbs forces your body to mobilize fat and this results in automatic fat loss and better health.

Feel free to mix and match the recipes you see in here and play around with them. Eating is supposed to be fun! Unfortunately, we've associated fun eating with unhealthy food. This doesn't have to be the case. The air fryer, combined with the Mediterranean diet, will make your mealtimes fun-filled again and full of taste. There's no grease and messy cleanups to deal with anymore. Are you excited yet? You should be! You're about to embark on a journey full of air fried goodness!

Salsa Stuffed Eggplants

Basic Recipe

Preparation Time: 15 minutes

Cooking Time: 25 minutes

Servings: 2

Ingredients

- 1 large eggplant
- teaspoons olive oil, divided
- teaspoons fresh lemon juice, divided
- cherry tomatoes, quartered
- tablespoons tomato salsa
- ½ tablespoon fresh parsley
- Salt and ground black pepper, as requiredDirections:

1 Set the temperature of air fryer to 390 degrees F. Grease an air fryer basket.

2 Place eggplant into the prepared air fryer basket.

3 Air fry for about 15 minutes

4 Remove from air fryer and cut the eggplant in half lengthwise.

5 Drizzle with the eggplant halves evenly with one teaspoon of oil.

6 Now, set the temperature of air fryer to 355 degrees F. Grease the air fryer basket.

7 Arrange eggplant into the prepared air fryer basket, cut-side up.

8 Air fry for another 10 minutes

9 Remove eggplant from the air fryer and set aside for about 5 minutes 10 Carefully, scoop out the flesh, leaving about ¼-inch away from edges.

11 Drizzle with the eggplant halves with one teaspoon of lemon juice.

12 Transfer the eggplant flesh into a bowl.

13 Add the tomatoes, salsa, parsley, salt, black pepper, remaining oil, and lemon juice and mix well.

14 Stuff the eggplant haves with salsa mixture and serve.

Nutrition: Calories 192 Carbs 33.8g Protein 6.9g Fat 6.1g

Sesame Seeds Bok Choy

Basic Recipe

Preparation Time: 10 minutes

Cooking Time: 6 minutes

Servings: 4

Ingredients

bunches baby bok choy, bottoms removed and leaves separated

Olive oil cooking spray

1 teaspoon garlic powder

1 teaspoon sesame seeds

Directions:

1 Set the temperature of air fryer to 325 degrees F.

2 Arrange bok choy leaves into the air fryer basket in a single layer.

3 Spray with the cooking spray and sprinkle with garlic powder.

4 Air fry for about 5-6 minutes, shaking after every 2 minutes

5 Remove from air fryer and transfer the bok choy onto serving plates.

6 Garnish with sesame seeds and serve hot.

Nutrition: Calories 26 Carbs 4g Protein 2.5g Fat 0.7g

Basil Tomatoes

Basic Recipe

Preparation Time: 10 minutes

Cooking Time: 10 minutes

Servings: 2

Ingredients

tomatoes, halved

Olive oil cooking spray

Salt and ground black pepper, as required

1 tablespoon fresh basil, chopped

Directions:

1 Set the temperature of air fryer to 320 degrees F. Grease an air fryer basket.

2 Spray the tomato halves evenly with cooking spray and sprinkle with salt, black pepper and basil.

3 Arrange tomato halves into the prepared air fryer basket, cut sides up.

4 Air-fry it for about 10 minutes or until desired doneness.

5 Remove from air fryer and transfer the tomatoes onto serving plates.

6 Serve warm.

Nutrition: Calories 22 Carbs 4.8g Protein 1.1g Fat 4.8g

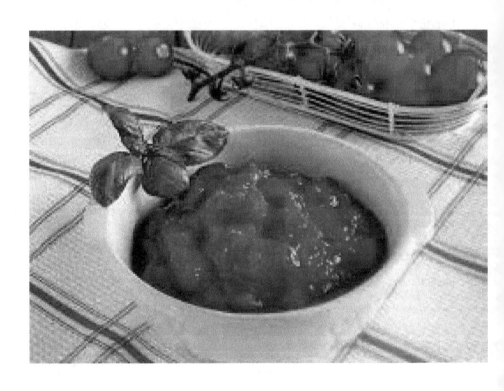

Overloaded Tomatoes

Basic Recipe

Preparation Time: 15 minutes

Cooking Time: 22 minutes

Servings: 4

Ingredients

tomatoes

1 teaspoon olive oil

1 carrot, peeled and finely chopped

1 onion, chopped

1 cup frozen peas, thawed 1 garlic clove, minced cups cold cooked rice

1 tablespoon soy sauce

Directions:

1 Cut the top of each tomato and scoop out pulp and seeds. In a skillet, heat oil over low heat and sauté the carrot, onion, garlic, and peas for about 2 minutes

2 Stir in the soy sauce and rice and remove from heat. Set the temperature of air fryer to 355 degrees F. Grease an air fryer basket.

3 Stuff each tomato with the rice mixture.

4 Arrange tomatoes into the prepared air fryer basket.

5 Air fry for about 20 minutes

6 Remove from air fryer and transfer the tomatoes onto a serving platter.

7 Set aside to cool slightly.

8 Serve warm.

Nutrition: Calories 421 Carbs 89.1g Protein 10.5g Fat 2.2g

Sweet & Spicy Cauliflower

Basic Recipe

Preparation Time: 15 minutes

Cooking Time: 30 minutes

Servings: 4

Ingredients

1 head cauliflower, cut into florets ¾ cup onion, thinly sliced garlic cloves, finely sliced 1½ tablespoons soy sauce

1 tablespoon hot sauce

1 tablespoon rice vinegar

1 teaspoon coconut sugar

Pinch of red pepper flakes Ground black pepper, as required scallions, chopped

Directions:

1 Set the temperature of air fryer to 350 degrees F. Grease an air fryer pan. Arrange cauliflower florets into the prepared air fryer pan in a single layer.

2 Air fry for about 10 minutes

3 Remove from air fryer and stir in the onions.

4 Air fry for another 10 minutes

5 Remove from air fryer and stir in the garlic.

6 Air fry for 5 more minutes

7 Meanwhile, in a bowl, mix well soy sauce, hot sauce, vinegar, coconut sugar, red pepper flakes, and black pepper.

8 Remove from the air fryer and stir in the sauce mixture.

9 Air fry for about 5 minutes

10 Remove from air fryer and transfer the cauliflower mixture onto serving plates. Garnish with scallions and serve.

Nutrition: Calories 72 Carbs 13.8g Protein 3.6g Fat 0.2g

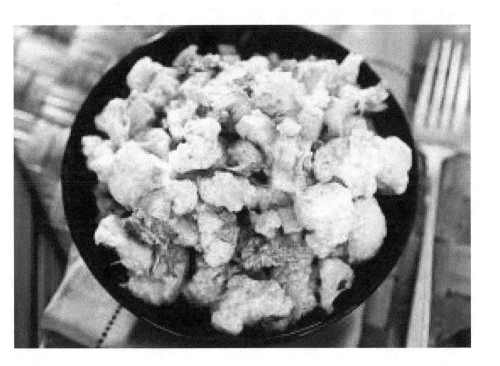

Spiced Butternut Squash

Basic Recipe

Preparation Time: 15 minutes

Cooking Time: 20 minutes

Servings: 4

Ingredients

1 medium butternut squash, peeled, seeded and cut into chunk teaspoons cumin seeds

1/8 teaspoon garlic powder

1/8 teaspoon chili flakes, crushed

Salt and ground black pepper, as required

1 tablespoon olive oil tablespoons pine nuts tablespoons fresh cilantro, chopped

Directions:

1 Set the temperature of air fryer to 375 degrees F. Grease an air fryer basket.

2 In a bowl, mix together the squash, spices, and oil.

3 Arrange butternut squash chunks into the prepared fryer basket.

4 Air fry it for about 20 minutes, flipping occasionally.

5 Remove from air fryer and transfer the squash chunks onto serving plates.

6 Garnish with pine nuts and cilantro.

7 Serve.

Nutrition: Calories 165 Carbs 27.6g Protein 3.1g Fat 6.9g

Spicy Potatoes

Basic Recipe

Preparation Time: 10 minutes

Cooking Time: 20 minutes

Servings: 6

Ingredients

1¾ pounds waxy potatoes, peeled and cubed

1 tablespoon olive oil

½ teaspoon ground cumin

½ teaspoon ground coriander

½ teaspoon paprika

Salt and freshly ground black pepper, as required

Directions:

1 In a large bowl of water, add the potatoes and set aside for about 30 minutes

2 Dry out the potatoes completely and dry with paper towels.

3 In a bowl, add the potatoes, oil, and spices and toss to coat well.

4 Set the temperature of air fryer to 355 degrees F. Grease an air fryer basket.

5 Arrange potato pieces into the prepared air fryer basket in a single layer.

6 Air fry for about 20 minutes

7 Remove from air fryer and transfer the potato pieces onto serving plates.

8 Serve hot.

Nutrition: Calories 113 Fat 2.5g Carbs 21g Protein 2.3g

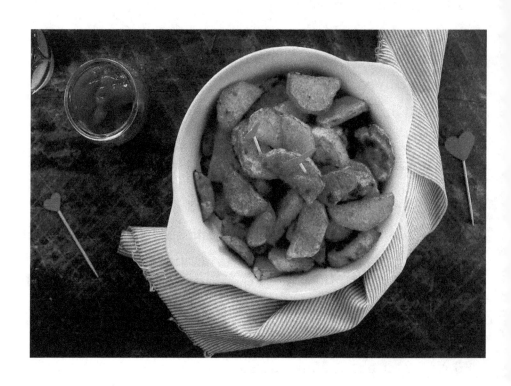

Crispy Kale Chips

Basic Recipe

Preparation Time: 5 minutes

Cooking Time: 7 minutes

Servings: 3

Ingredients

• 3 cups kale leaves, stems removed

• 1 tablespoon olive oil

• Salt and pepper, to tasteDirections:

1 In a bowl, combine all of the ingredients. Toss to coat the kale leaves with oil, salt, and pepper.

2 Arrange the kale leaves on the double layer rack and insert inside the air fryer.

3 Close the air fryer and cook for 7 minutes at 3700F.

4 Allow to cool before serving.

Nutrition: Calories 48 Carbs 1.4g Protein 0.7g Fat 4.8g

Grilled Buffalo Cauliflower

Basic Recipe

Preparation Time: 5 minutes

Cooking Time: 5 minutes

Servings: 1

Ingredients

1 cup cauliflower florets

Cooking oil spray

Salt and pepper, to taste

½ cup buffalo sauce

Directions

1 Place the cauliflower florets in a bowl and spray with cooking oil. Season it with salt and pepper.

2 Toss to coat.

3 Place the grill pan in the air fryer and add the cauliflower florets.

4 Close the lid and cook for 5 minutes at 3900F.

5 Once cooked, place in a bowl and pour the buffalo sauce over the top. Toss to coat.

Nutrition: Calories 25 Fat 0.1g Carbs 5.3g Protein 2g

Barbacoa Beef

Basic Recipe

Preparation Time: 15 minutes

Cooking Time: 1hour and 20 minutes

Servings: 10

Ingredients

2/3 cup beer cloves garlic chipotles in adobo sauce 1 tsp. black pepper

1/4 tsp. ground cloves

1 tbsp. olive oil

3-pound beef chuck roast, 2-inch chunks bay leaves 1 onion, chopped oz. chopped green chilies 1/4 cup lime juice tbsp. apple cider vinegar 1 tbsp. ground cumin 1 tbsp. dried Mexican oregano tsp. salt

Directions:

1-Puree beer, garlic, chipotles, onion, green chilies, lime juice, vinegar, and seasonings.

2- Sauté roast in oil.

3-Add the bay leaves and pureed sauce.

4- Cook on High Pressure for 60 minutes

5-Discard the leaves.

6- Shred beef and serve with sauce.

Nutrition: Calories 520 kcal Fat 23g Carbs 56 g Protein 31g

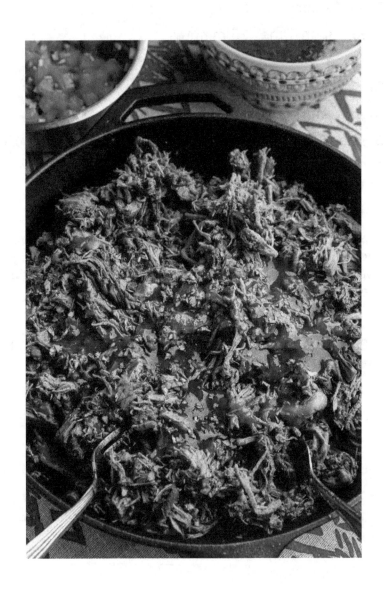

Maple Smoked Brisket

Basic Recipe

Preparation Time: 15 minutes

Cooking Time: 1hour and 20 minutes

Servings: 4

Ingredients

 beef brisket

1 tbsp. maple sugar

c. bone broth or stock of choice 1 tbsp. liquid smoke fresh thyme sprigs tsp. smoked sea salt 1 tsp. black pepper

1 tsp. mustard powder

1 tsp. onion powder

½ tsp. smoked paprika

Directions:

1 Coat the brisket with all spices and sugar.

2 Sauté brisket in oil for 3 minutes

3 Add broth, liquid smoke, and thyme to the Air fryer and cover.

4 Cook at High Pressure for 50 minutes

5 Remove brisket.

6 Sauté sauce for 10 minutes

7 Serve sliced brisket with any whipped vegetable and sauce.

Nutrition: Calories 1671 kcal Fat 43g Carbs 98 g Protein 56g

Philly Cheesesteak Sandwiches

Basic Recipe

Preparation Time: 5 minutes

Cooking Time: 30 minutes

Servings: 8

Ingredients

 3-pound beef top sirloin steak, sliced onions, julienned

1 can condensed French onion soup, undiluted garlic cloves, minced

1 package Italian salad dressing mix tsp. beef base 1/2 tsp. pepper large red peppers, julienned 1/2 cup pickled pepper rings hoagie buns, split slices provolone cheese

Directions:

1 Combine the first 7 ingredients in the pressure cooker. Adjust to pressure-cook on High for 10 minutes. Add peppers and pepper rings. Pressure-cook on High for 5 minutes

2 Put beef, cheese, and vegetables on bun bottoms. Broil 1-2 minutes and serve.

Nutrition: Calories 4852 kcal Fat 67g Carbs 360 g Protein 86g

Pot Roast and Potatoes

Basic Recipe

Preparation Time: 15 minutes

Cooking Time: 1 hour and 15 minutes

Servings: 8

Ingredients

tbsp. all-purpose flour 1 tbsp. kosher salt lb. chuck roast 1 tbsp. black pepper

c. low-sodium beef broth

1/2 c. red wine

1 lb. baby potatoes, halved 1 tbsp. Worcestershire sauce

carrots, sliced

1 onion, chopped

1 tbsp. extra-virgin olive oil cloves garlic, minced 1 tsp. thyme, chopped tsp. rosemary, chopped tbsp. tomato paste

Directions:

1 Coat chuck roast with pepper and salt.

2 Sauté the beef for 5 minutes on each side then set aside.

3 Cook onion for 5 minutes

4 Add herbs, garlic, and tomato paste and cook for 1 minute.

5 Add four and wine and cook for 2 minutes

6 Add Worcestershire sauce, broth, carrots, potatoes, salt and pepper.

7 Put beef on top of the mixture

8 High-Pressure Cook for an hour and serve.

Nutrition: Calories 3274 kcal Fat 42 g Carbs 286 g Protein 78 g

Butter Chicken

Intermediate Recipe

Preparation Time: 10 minutes

Cooking Time: 1hour and 10 minutes

Servings: 6

Ingredients

1 tbsp. vegetable oil

1 tbsp. butter 1 onion, diced tsp. grated ginger 1 tsp. ground cumin

1/2 tsp. turmeric

1/ 2 tsp. kosher salt

½ tsp. black pepper 3/4 c. heavy cream cloves garlic, chopped oz. tomato paste lb. boneless chicken thighs, 1" pieces

1 tbsp. garam masala

1 tsp. paprika

1 tbsp. sugar

Directions:

1 Sauté the onion, ginger, and garlic in oil and butter

2 Add tomato paste and cook for 3 minutes

3 Add ½ cup water, chicken, and spices to the Pot.

4 Pressure Cook on High for 5 minutes

5 Add heavy cream.

6 Serve with rice, naan, yogurt, and cilantro.

Nutrition: Calories 3841 Fat 100g Carbs 244g Protein 150g

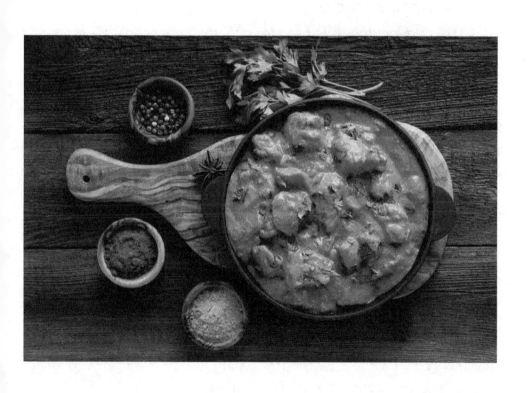

Curried Chicken Meatball Wraps

Basic Recipe

Preparation Time: 5 minutes

Cooking Time: 15 minutes

Servings: 12

Ingredients

1 egg, beaten

1 onion, chopped

1/2 cup Rice Krispies

1/4 cup golden raisins 1/4 cup minced cilantro tsp. curry powder

1/2 tsp. salt

Boston lettuce leaves

1 carrot, shredded

1/2 cup chopped salted peanuts 1-pound lean ground chicken

tbsp. olive oil

1 cup plain yogurt

Directions:

1 Mix the first 7 ingredients.

2 Shape mixture into 24 balls. 3 Sauté meatballs on medium with oil

4 Add water to pot.

5 Put meatballs on the trivet in the pressure cooker.

6 Pressure-cook on High for 7 minutes

 7 Mix yogurt and cilantro.

8 Place 2 teaspoons sauce and 1 meatball in each lettuce leaf; top with remaining ingredients and serve. Nutrition: Calories 2525 Fat 80g Carbs 225g Protein 120g

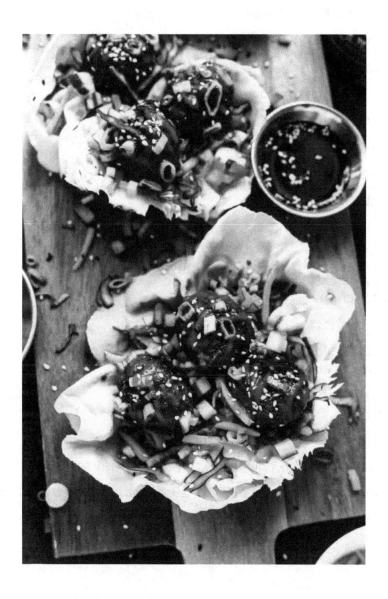

Fall-Off-The-Bone Chicken

Intermediate Recipe

Preparation Time: 10 minutes

Cooking Time: 1hour and 10 minutes

Servings: 4

Ingredients

1 tbsp. packed brown sugar

1 tbsp. chili powder

1 tbsp. smoked paprika

1 tsp. chopped thyme leaves

¼ tbsp. kosher salt

¼ tbsp. black pepper

1 whole small chicken

1 tbsp. extra-virgin olive oil 2/3 c. low-sodium chicken broth tbsp. chopped parsley

Directions:

1 Coat chicken with brown sugar, chili powder, sugar, pepper, paprika, and thyme.

2 Sauté chicken in oil for 3-4 minutes 3   Pour broth in the Pot.

4 Pressure Cook on High for 25 minutes

5 Garnish sliced chicken with parsley and serve.

Nutrition: Calories 1212 Fat 10g Carbs 31g Protein 15g

White Chicken Chili

Basic Recipe

Preparation Time: 5 minutes

Cooking Time: 30 minutes

Servings: 6

Ingredients

1 tbsp. vegetable oil

1 red bell pepper, diced

• oz. condensed cream of chicken soup

tbsp. shredded Cheddar cheese green onions, sliced 1 cup Kernel corn 1 tbsp. chili powder

oz. (2) boneless, skinless chicken breast oz. white cannellini beans

1 cup Chunky Salsa

Directions:

Sauté pepper, corn, and chili powder in oil for 2 minutes Season chicken with salt and pepper.

Layer the beans, salsa, water, chicken, and soup over the corn mixture. Pressure Cook on High for 4 minutes Shred chicken and return to pot.

Serve topped with cheese and green onions.

Nutrition: Calories 1848 Fat 70g Carbs 204g Protein 90g

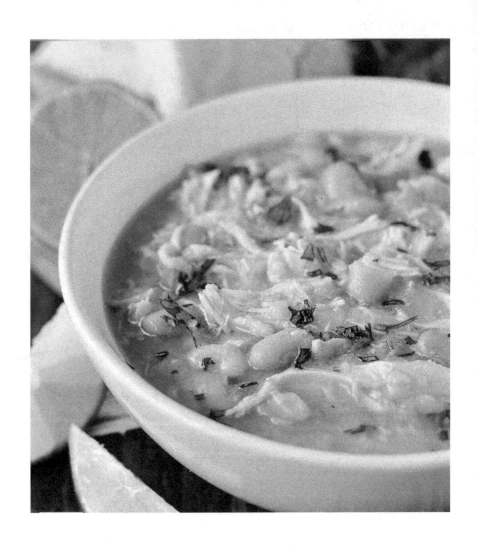

Coconut Curry Vegetable Rice Bowls

Basic Recipe

Preparation Time: 5 minutes

Cooking Time: 40minutes

Servings: 6

Ingredients

2/3 cup uncooked brown rice

1 tsp. curry powder

3/4 tsp. salt divided

1 cup chopped green onion

1 cup sliced red bell pepper

1 tbsp. grated ginger

1 1/2 tbsp. sugar

1 cup matchstick carrots 1 cup chopped red cabbage oz. sliced water chestnuts oz. no salt added chickpeas oz. coconut milk

Directions:

·1   Add rice, water, curry powder, and 1/4 tsp. of the salt in the Air fryer. Pressure Cook for 15 minutes. Sauté for 2 minutes and serve.

Nutrition: Calories 1530 Fat 110g Carbs 250g Protein 80g

Egg Roll in a Bowl

Basic Recipe

Preparation Time: 5 minutes

Cooking Time: 20 minutes

Servings: 4

Ingredients

1/3 cup low-sodium soy sauce tbsp. sesame oil

1 cup matchstick cut carrots 1 bunch green onions, sliced bags coleslaw mix 1 lb. ground chicken tbsp. sesame seeds cloves garlic, minced oz. shiitake mushrooms, sliced

1 1/2 cups chicken broth

Directions:

1 Add sesame oil, ground chicken, soy sauce, garlic, chicken broth and mushrooms to Air fryer.

2 Cook for 2 minutes on High Pressure.

3 Add in coleslaw mix and carrots.

4 Let sit for 5 minutes

5 Serve with sesame seeds and green onions.

Nutrition: Calories 3451 Fat 130g Carbs 301g Protein 150g

Frittata Provencal

Basic Recipe

Preparation Time: 5 minutes

Cooking Time: 45 minutes

Servings: 6 Ingredients

eggs

1 tsp. minced thyme

1 tsp. hot pepper sauce

1/2 tsp. salt

1/4 tsp. pepper oz. goat cheese, divided

1/2 cup chopped sun-dried tomatoes

1 tbsp. olive oil

1 potato, peeled and sliced

1 onion, sliced

1/2 tsp. smoked paprika

Directions:

1-Sauté potato, paprika, and onion in oil for 5-7 minutes

2 Transfer potato mixture to a greased baking dish.

3 Pour the first 6 ingredients over potato mixture.

4 Cover baking dish with foil.

5 Add water and trivet to pot.

6 Use a foil sling to lower the dish onto the trivet.

7 Adjust to pressure-cook on high for 35 minutes and serve.

Nutrition: Calories 2554 Fat 70g Carbs 190g Protein 80g

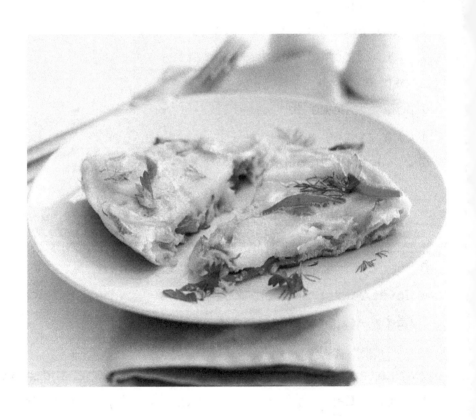

Ramekin Eggs

Basic Recipe

Preparation Time: 2 minutes

Cooking Time: 3minutes

Servings: 2

Ingredients

1 tbsp. ghee, plus more for greasing

cups mushrooms, chopped

¼ tsp. salt

1 tbsp. chives, chopped eggs tbsp. heavy cream

Directions:

1-Sauté mushrooms with ghee and salt until tender.

2 Put mushrooms into greased ramekins.

3 Add chives, egg, and cream.

4 Add water, trivet, and ramekins to pot.

5 Pressure Cook on Low for 1-2 minutes

 6 Serve with freshly toasted bread.

Nutrition: Calories 703 Fat 5g Carbs 20g Protein 7g

Easter Ham

Basic Recipe

Preparation Time: 5 minutes

Cooking Time: 15 minutes

Servings: 8

Ingredients

1/2 c. orange marmalade

¼ tsp. black pepper

1 (4-6 lb.) fully cooked, spiral, bone-in ham

1/4 c. brown sugar 1/4 c. orange juice tbsp. Dijon mustard

Directions:

1 Mix marmalade, brown sugar, orange juice, Dijon, and black pepper.

2 Coat ham with glaze.

3 Cook on Meat for 15 minutes

4 Serve ham with more glaze from the Pot.

Nutrition: Calories 3877 Fat 80g Carbs 207g Protein 100g

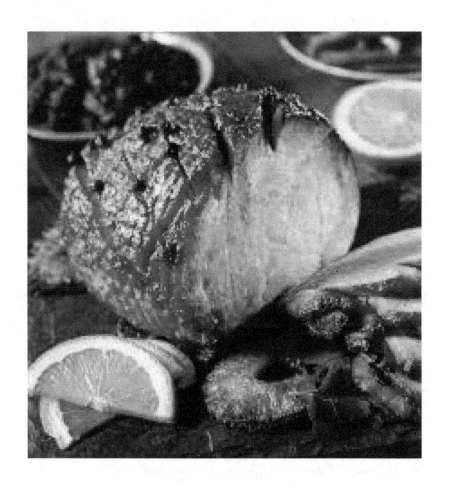

Korean Lamb Chops

Intermediate Recipe

Preparation Time: 10 minutes

Cooking Time: 50minutes

Servings: 6

Ingredients

lbs. Lamb chops 1/2 tsp. Red pepper powder tbsp. granulated sugar 1 tbsp. curry powder 1/2 tbsp. soy sauce tbsp. rice wine tbsp. garlic, minced 1 tsp. ginger, minced bay leaves 1 cup carrots, diced cups onions, diced 1 cup celery, diced tbsp. Korean red pepper paste tbsp. ketchup tbsp. Corn syrup 1/2 tbsp. sesame oil

1/2 tsp. cinnamon powder

1 tsp. sesame seeds

1 tsp. black pepper

1/3 cup Asian pear ground

1/3 cup onion powder

1/2 tbsp. Green plum extract

1 cup red wine

Directions:

1 Put all ingredients except cilantro and green onions into the Air fryer.

2 Pressure Cook for 20 minutes 3   Sauté until sauce is thickened.

4 Add water and lamb on trivet to pot.

5 Broil at 400°F for 5 minutes

6 Serve with chopped cilantro and green onions.

Nutrition: Calories 2728 Fat 220g Carbs 551g Protein 250g

Air Fryer Chicken Kabobs

Basic Recipe

Preparation Time: 15 minutes

Cooking Time: 15 minutes

Servings: 2

Ingredients

Chicken breasts, chopped

Mushrooms cut into halves

⅓ Cup honey

⅓ Cup Soy sauce -

1 teaspoon Pepper, crushed

1 teaspoon Sesame seeds

Bell peppers, in different colors

 Cooking oil spray as required

Directions:

1 Cut the chicken breasts into small cubes, wash and pat dry. Rub little pepper and salt over the chicken. Sprits some oil on it. In a small bowl, combine honey and soy sauce thoroughly.

2 Add the sesame seeds into the mix. Drive in chicken, bell peppers and mushrooms onto the skewers.

3 Set the air fryer at 170 degrees Celsius and preheat.

4 Drizzle with the kabobs with the honey and soy sauce mixture.

5 Put all the skewed chicken kabobs into the air fryer basket and cook for 20 minutes

6 Rotate the skewer intermittently in between.

7 Serve hot.

Nutrition: Calories 392 Fal 5g Carbs 65.4g Protein 6.7g

Chicken Fried Rice in Air Fryer

Basic Recipe

Preparation Time: 20 minutes

Cooking Time: 20 minutes

Servings: 4

Ingredients

cups cooked cold white rice 1 cup chicken cooked & diced

1 cup carrots and peas, frozen

1 tablespoon vegetable oil

1 tablespoon soy sauce

½ cup onion

¼ teaspoon salt

Directions:

1 In a large bowl, put the cooked cold rice.

2 Stir in soy sauce and vegetable oil.

3 Now add the frozen carrots and peas, diced chicken, diced onion, salt and combine.

4 Transfer the rice mixture into the mix.

5 Take a non-stick pan which you can comfortably place in the air fryer and transfer the complete rice mixture into the pan.

6 Place the pan in the air fryer.

7 Set the temperature at 180 degree Celsius and timer for 20 minutes

8 Remove the pan after the set time elapse.

9 Serve hot.

Nutrition: Calories 618 Fat 5.5g Carbs 116.5g Protein 21.5g

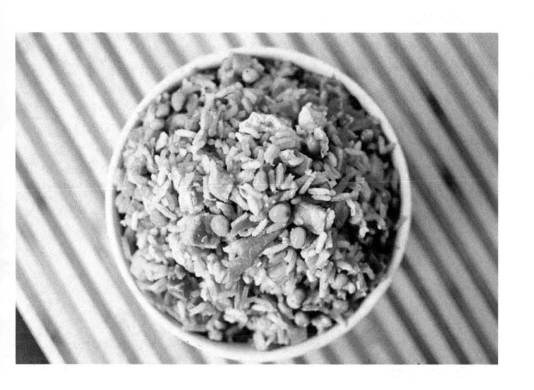

Air Fried Chicken Tikkas

Basic Recipe

Preparation Time: 10 minutes

Cooking Time: 15 minutes

Servings: 4

Ingredients For marinade:

1¼ pounds chicken, bones cut into small bite size

¼ pound cherry tomatoes

1 cup yogurt

1 tablespoon ginger garlic paste (fresh) bell peppers, 1" cut size tablespoons chili powder tablespoons cumin powder 1 tablespoon turmeric powder tablespoons coriander powder

1 teaspoon garam masala powder

teaspoons olive oil Salt – to taste

For garnishing:

1 lemon, cut into half

⅓ cup Coriander, fresh, chopped

1 medium Onion, nicely sliced Mint leaves, fresh – few

Directions:

1 In a large bowl mix all the marinade ingredients and coat it thoroughly on the chicken pieces.

2 Cover the bowl and set aside for 2 hours minimum. If you can refrigerate overnight, it can give better marinade effect.

3 Thread the chicken in the skewers along with bell peppers and tomatoes alternately.

4 Preheat your air fryer at 200 degrees Celsius.

5 Spread an aluminum liner on the air fryer basket and arrange the skewers on it.

6 Set the timer for 15 minutes and grill it.

7 Turn the skewer intermittently for an even grilling.

8 Once done, put into a plate and garnish with the given ingredients before serving.

Nutrition: Calories 400 Fat 20g Carbs 17.4g Protein 46.9g

Nashville Hot Chicken in Air Fryer

Basic Recipe

Preparation Time: 10 minutes

Cooking Time: 27 minutes

Servings: 4

Ingredients

pounds chicken with bones, 8 pieces tablespoons vegetable oil cups all-purpose flour 1 cup buttermilk tablespoons paprika 1 teaspoon onion powder 1 teaspoon garlic powder 1 teaspoon ground black pepper teaspoons salt

For Hot sauce:

1 tablespoon cayenne pepper

¼ cup vegetable oil 1 teaspoon salt slices white bread

Dill pickle, as required

Directions:

1 Clean and wash chicken thoroughly, pat dry and keep ready aside.

2 In a bowl, whisk buttermilk and eggs.

3 Combine garlic powder, black pepper, paprika, onion powder, All-purpose flour and salt in a bowl.

4 Now dip the chicken in the egg and buttermilk and put in the second bowl marinade bowl and toss to get an even coating. Maybe you need to repeat the process twice for a better coat.

5 After that spray some vegetable oil and keep aside.

6 Before cooking the chicken, pre-heat the fryer at 190 degrees Celsius.

7 Brush vegetable oil on the fry basket before start cooking.

8 Now place the coated chicken in the air fryer at 190 degrees Celsius and set the timer for 20 minutes. Do not crowd the air fryer. It would be better if you can do the frying in 2 batches.

9 Keep the flipping the chicken intermittently for even frying.

10 Once the set timer elapsed, remove the chicken to a plate and keep it there without covering.

11 Now start the second batch. Do the same process.

12 After 20 minutes, reduce the temperature to 170 degrees Celsius and place the first batch of chicken over the second batch, which is already in the air fry basket.

13 Fry it again for another 7 minutes

14 While the chicken is air frying, make the hot sauce.

15 In a bowl mix salt and cayenne pepper thoroughly.

16 In a small saucepan, heat some vegetable oil.

17 When the oil becomes hot add the spice mix and continue stirring to become smooth.

18 While serving, place the chicken over the white bread and spread the hot sauce over the chicken.

19 Use dill pickle to top it.

20 Serve hot.

Nutrition: Calories 1013 Fat 22.2g Carbs 53.9g Protein 140.7g

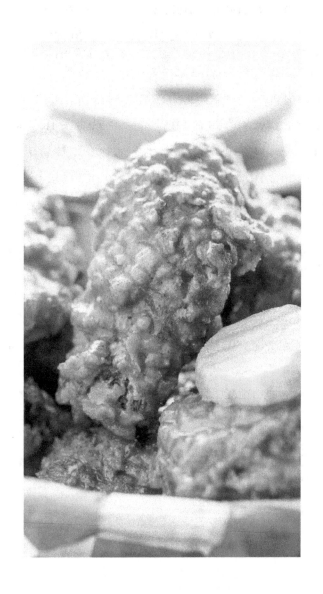

Air Fryer Panko Breaded Chicken Parmesan

Basic Recipe

Preparation Time: 10 minutes

Cooking Time: 20 minutes

Servings: 4

Ingredients

ounces chicken breasts, skinless

1 cup panko bread crumbs

⅛ cup egg whites

½ cup parmesan cheese, shredded

½ cup mozzarella cheese, grated

¾ cup marinara sauce

½ teaspoon salt

1 teaspoon ground pepper teaspoons italian seasoning Cooking spray, as required

Directions:

1 Cut each chicken breast into halves to make 4 breast pieces. Wash and pat dry.

2 Place the chicken in a chopping board and pound to flatten.

3 Sprits the air fryer basket with cooking oil.

4 Set the temperature of air fryer to 200 degrees Celsius and preheat.

5 In a large bowl, mix cheese, panko breadcrumbs, and seasoning ingredients.

6 Put the egg white in a large bowl.

7 Dip the pounded chicken into the egg whites and dredge into breadcrumb mixture.

8 Now place the coated chicken into the air fryer basket and spray some cooking oil.

9 Start cooking the chicken breasts for 7 minutes

10 Dress on top of the chicken breasts with shredded mozzarella and marinara sauce.

11 Continue cooking for another 3 minutes and remove for serving when the cheese starts to melt. Nutrition: Calories 347 Fat 15g Carbs 7.4g Protein 37g

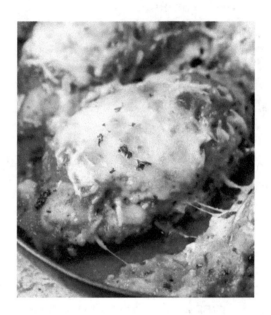

Air Fryer Rosemary Turkey

Basic Recipe

Preparation Time: 5 minutes

Cooking Time: 30 minutes

Servings: 6

Ingredients

2½ pounds turkey breast teaspoons fresh rosemary, chopped

¼ cup olive oil

cloves garlic, minced

1 teaspoon crushed pepper

¼ cup maple syrup

1 tablespoon ground mustard

1 tablespoon butter

1½ teaspoon salt

Directions:

1 Combine thoroughly, minced garlic, olive oil, shredded rosemary, pepper and salt in medium bowl.

2 Rub the herb seasoning and oil all over the turkey breast loins.

3 Cover and refrigerate for at least 2 hours for better marinade effect.

4 Before cooking, allow it to thaw for half an hour.

5 Spray some cooking oil on the air fryer basket and place the turkey breast on it.

6 Set the temperature at 200 degrees Celsius for 20 minutes

7 Flip the turkey breast intermittently.

8 While cooking in progress, melt a tablespoon of butter in a microwave oven.

9 Stir in mustard powder and maple syrup in the melted butter.

10 Pour the sauce mix over the turkey breast and continue cooking for another 10 minutes 11   After the cooking is over, slice it for serving.

Nutrition: Calories 292 Fat 13.5g Carbs 9.5g Protein 15g

Air Fryer Lamb Chops

Basic Recipe

Preparation Time: 5 minutes

Cooking Time: 30 minutes

Servings: 2

Ingredients

lamb chops

½ tablespoon oregano, fresh, coarsely chopped

1½ tablespoons olive oil

1 teaspoon black pepper, ground

1 clove garlic

½ teaspoon salt

Directions:

1 Set the air fryer temperature to 200 degrees Celsius.

2 Spray olive on garlic clove and place it in the air fryer basket.

3 Bake it for 12 minutes

4 Combine herbs with pepper, olive oil, and salt.

5 Rub half of the mix over the lamb chops and set aside for 3 minutes

6 Remove the roasted garlic clove from the air fryer.

7 Set the temperature at 200 degrees Celsius and preheat the air fryer.

8 Layer the lamb chops into the air fryer basket and cook for 5 minutes or until it becomes brown.

9 Do not roast the lambs altogether by overlapping one over the other. You can do the roasting in batches.

10 After finish roasting, squeeze the garlic into the herb sauce.

11 Add some more salt and pepper if required.

12 Serve the dish along with garlic sauce.

Nutrition: Calories 97 Fat 10.7g Carbs 1.3g Protein 0.3g

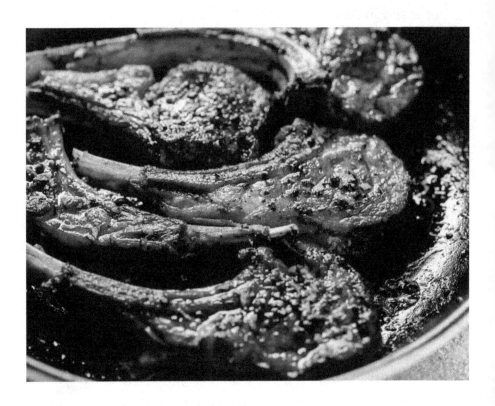

Air Fried Shrimp and Sauce

Basic Recipe

Preparation Time: 10 minutes

Cooking Time: 20 minutes

Servings: 4

Ingredients

1 pound shrimps

½ cup all-purpose flour

1 egg white

¾ cup panko breadcrumbs tablespoons chicken seasoning

1 teaspoon paprika

1 teaspoon pepper

½ teaspoon salt

Cooking spray, as required To make the sauce:

⅓ cup of greek yogurt, non-fat ¼ cup sweet chili sauce tablespoons sriracha

Directions:

1 Peel, devein, clean, wash and pat dry the shrimps.

2 Marinate the shrimps by using the seasoning.

3 Put egg white, all-purpose flour and breadcrumbs in three separate bowls.

4 Set the temperature to 200 degree Celsius and preheat the air fryer.

5 Dip the seasoned shrimp in flour, then in the egg white and finally dredge in the breadcrumbs.

6 Sprits cooking oil on the coated shrimp.

7 Put the shrimps in the air fryer basket and cook for 4 minutes

8 Flip the shrimps and cook further 4 minutes

9 For making the sauce, blend all the sauce ingredients in a medium bowl thoroughly.

10 Serve the shrimps along with the sauce.

Nutrition: Calories 318 Fat 6.7g Carbs 30.7g Protein 31.3g

Air Fryer Italian Meatball

Basic Recipe

Preparation Time: 6minutes

Cooking Time: 15 minutes

Servings: 6 Ingredients

pounds ground beef eggs

1¼ cup bread crumbs

¼ cup fresh parsley, chopped

1 teaspoon dried oregano

¼ cup parmigiano reggiano, grated

1 teaspoon light cooking oil

Salt to taste

Pepper, as required

Tomato sauce, for serving

Directions:

1 In a mixing bowl put the meat and all ingredients except the cooking oil.

2 Hand mix all the ingredients. Once the mix blended thoroughly, make a small ball with your hand. The given quantity is enough to make 24 balls.

3 Spread a liner paper in the air fryer basket and lightly coat it with cooking oil.

4 Place the bowls in the air fryer basket without overlapping one another.

5 Set the temperature to 200 degrees Celsius and cook for 12-14 minutes until its side becomes brown.

6 Once the sides become brown, turn the balls and cook for another 5 minutes

7 Serve hot along with tomato sauce.

Nutrition: Calories 405 Fat 13.1g Carbs 16.5g Protein 52.1g

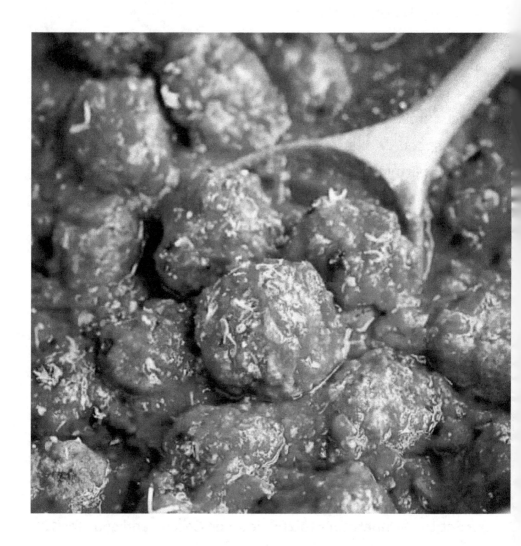

Air Fryer Coconut Milk Chicken

Basic Recipe

Preparation Time: 10 minutes

Cooking Time: 18 minutes

Servings: 6

Ingredients

1¾ pounds Chicken thighs with skin and bone -

Marinade:

cups coconut milk

teaspoons ground black pepper

1 teaspoon cayenne pepper, ground 1 teaspoon salt Seasoned flour:

1 tablespoon baking powder 1 tablespoon paprika powder cups all-purpose flour

1 tablespoon garlic powder

1 teaspoon salt

Directions:

1 Clean, wash the chicken thighs and pat dry.

2 Combine paprika, cayenne pepper, black pepper, salt in a large bowl.

3 Put chicken into it and toss to coat the ingredients.

4 Pour buttermilk until chicken covered.

5 Refrigerate the coated chicken for a minimum of 6 hours.

6 Set the air fryer temperature to 180 degrees Celsius.

7 In another bowl combine the seasoning flour such as baking powder, paprika, all-purpose flour, garlic powder, and salt.

8 Now take out the chicken from the refrigerator and thaw it for some time.

9 Dredge the chicken into the flour and remove excess flour by shaking off it.

10 Place the coated chicken into the air fryer basket.

11 Cook it for 8 minutes

12 After 8 minutes flip the chicken pieces and cook for another 10 minutes

13 Transfer the cooked chicken onto a paper towel, so that the excess juice can dry out quickly.

14 Serve hot.

Nutrition: Calories 384 Fat 21.7g Carbs 39.2g Protein 12.1g

Air Fryer Cauliflower Rice

Basic Recipe

Preparation Time: 10 minutes

Cooking Time: 20 minutes

Servings: 3

Ingredients

Segment - 1

½ firm tofu ½ cup onion, chopped

tablespoons low sodium soy sauce

1 cup carrot diced

½ teaspoon turmeric powder

Segment – 2 cups cauliflower rice ½ cup frozen peas tablespoons low sodium soy sauce

1½ teaspoons sesame oil, toasted

1 tablespoon rice vinegar

1 tablespoon ginger, grated

½ cup broccoli, finely chopped cloves garlic, minced

Directions:

1 Crumble tofu in a large bowl. Toss the crumbled tofu with sector 1 ingredients.

2 Set the air fryer temperature to 190 degree Celsius and cook for 10 minutes. Shake the air fryer basket 2-3 times during the cooking in progress.

3 In another large bowl, combine all the ingredients mentioned in the segment 2.

4 After 10 minutes of cooking, transfer the second segment ingredients over the cooked food. Shake the air basket tray and cook for 10 minutes at 190 degrees Celsius. Make sure to shake the air frycr basket intermittently for a better baking

result. When the cauliflower rice becomes tender, it is ready to serve.

5 Serve hot along with your favorite sauce.

Buttery Cod

Basic Recipe

Preparation Time: 5 minutes

Cooking Time: 15 minutes

Servings: 4

Ingredients

tbsp parsley, chopped tbsp butter, melted cherry tomatoes, halved 0.25 cup tomato sauce cod fillets, cubed

Directions:

1 Turn on the air fryer to 390 degrees.

2 Combine all of the ingredients and put them into a pan that works with the air fryer.

3 After 12 minutes of baking, you can divide this between the four bowls and enjoy.

Nutrition: Calories 232 Fat 8g Carbs 5g Protein 11g

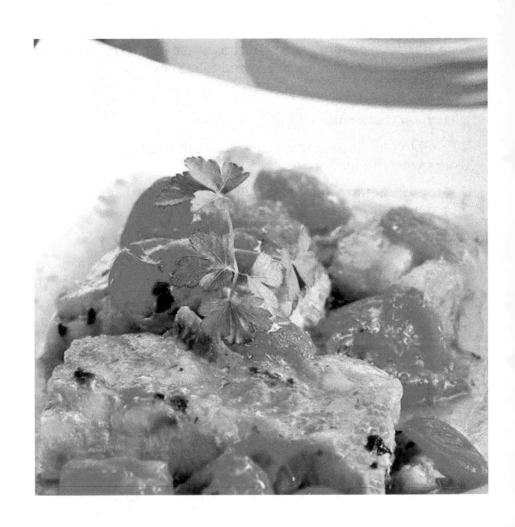

Creamy Chicken

Basic Recipe

Preparation Time: 5 minutes

Cooking Time: 15 minutes

Servings: 4

Ingredients

Pepper and salt

1 tsp olive oil

1 0.5 tsp sweet paprika 0.25 cup coconut cream chicken breasts, cubed

Directions:

1 Turn on the air fryer to 370 degrees. Prepare a frying pan that fits into the machine with some oil before adding the ingredients inside. Add this to the air fryer and let it bake. After 17 minutes, you can divide between the few plates and serve!

Nutrition: Calories 250 Fat 12g Carbs 5g Protein 11g

Mushroom and Turkey Stew

Basic Recipe

Preparation Time: 5 minutes

Cooking Time: 25 minutes

Servings: 4

Ingredients

Pepper and salt

1 tbsp parsley, chopped

0.25 cup tomato sauce

1 turkey breast cubed

0.5 lb. Brown mushrooms, sliced

Directions:

1 Turn on the air fryer to 350 degrees. Pick out a pan and mix the tomato sauce, pepper, salt, mushrooms, and turkey together. Add to the air fryer.

2 After 25 minutes, the stew is done—divides between four bowls and top with the parsley. Nutrition: Calories 220 Fat 12g Carbs 5g Protein 12g

Meatball Casserole

Basic Recipe

Preparation Time: 5 minutes

Cooking Time: 15 minutes

Servings: 6

Ingredients

1 tbsp thyme, chopped

0.25 cup parsley, chopped

0.33 lb turkey sausage

1 egg, beaten

0.66 lb ground beef tbsp olive oil 1 shallot, minced 1 tbsp Dijon mustard garlic cloves, minced tbsp whole milk

1 tbsp rosemary, chopped

Directions:

1 Turn on the air fryer to a High setting and then give it time to heat up with some oil inside.

2 Add the garlic and onions and cook for a few minutes to make soft.

3 Add the milk and bread crumbs to a bowl and then mix. Then add in the rest of the ingredients and set aside to soak.

4 Use this mixture, after five minutes, to prepare some small meatballs. Add these to the air fryer.

5 Turn the heat up to 400 degrees to cook. After 10 minutes, take the lid off and shake the basket. Cook another five minutes before serving.

Nutrition: Calories 168 Fat 11g Carbs 4g Protein 12g

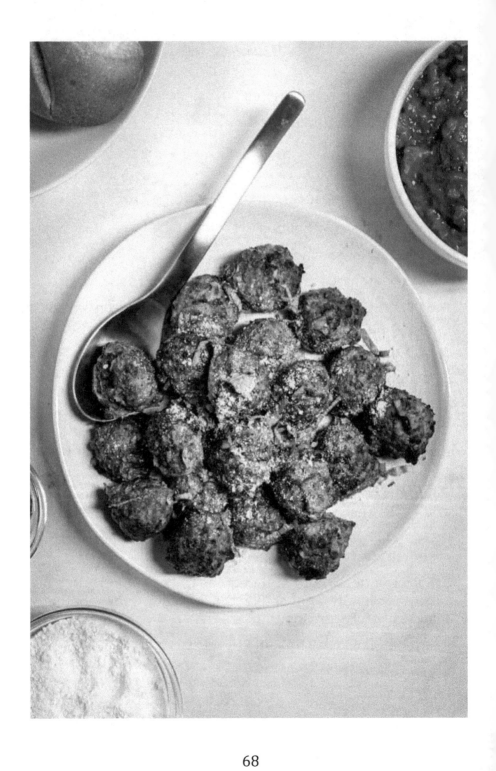

Herbed Lamb Rack

Basic Recipe

Preparation Time: 5 minutes

Cooking Time: 10 minutes

Servings: 2

Ingredients

tbsp olive oil 0.5 tsp pepper 1 tbsp dried thyme tbsp dried rosemary

0.5 tsp salt tsp garlic, minced

1 lb rack of lamb

Directions:

1 Turn on the air fryer to 400 degrees. In a bowl, combine the herbs and olive oil well.

2 Use this to coat the lamb before adding to the basket of the air fryer.

3 Close the lid, and then let this cook. Halfway through, you can shake the basket to make sure nothing sticks.

4 After ten minutes, take the lamb out and enjoy.

Nutrition: Calories 542 Fat 37g Carbs 3g Protein 45g

Baked Beef

Intermediate Recipe

Preparation Time: 10 minutes

Cooking Time: 60minutes

Servings: 5

Ingredients

1 bunch garlic cloves 1 bunch fresh herbs, mixed

sliced onions Olive oil lbs beef celery sticks, chopped carrots, chopped Directions:

1 Great up a pan and then add the herbs, olive oil, beef roast, and vegetables inside.

2 Turn the air fryer on to 400 degrees and place the pan inside. Let this heat up and close the lid.

3 After an hour of cooking, open the lid and then serve this right away.

Nutrition: Calories 306 Fat 21g Carbs 10g Protein 32g

Chicken Wings

Basic Recipe

Preparation Time: 5 minutes

Cooking Time: 25 minutes

Servings: 2

Ingredients

tbsp. chives 0.5 tbsp. salt

1 tbsp lime

0.5 tbsp ginger, chopped

1 tbsp garlic, minced 1 tbsp chili paste tbsp honey 0.5 tbsp cornstarch

1 tbsp soy sauce

Oil chicken wings

Directions:

1 Dry the chicken and then cover it with spray. Add into the air fryer that is preheated to 400 degrees.

2 Let this cook for a bit. During that time, add the rest of the ingredients to a bowl and set aside.

3 After 25 minutes, the chicken is done. Add the chicken into a bowl and top with the sauce. Sprinkle the chives on top and serve.

Nutrition: Calories 81 Fat 5g Carbs 0g Protein 8g

Sesame Chicken

Basic Recipe

Preparation Time: 5 minutes

Cooking Time: 50minutes

Servings: 4

Ingredients

Soy sauce

Pepper

Salt

Olive oil

Breadcrumbs

Egg

1 lb. Chicken breast

Directions:

1 Slice the chicken into fillets and add to the bowl with the sesame and soy sauce. Let this marinate for half an hour. Beat the eggs and then pass the chicken through it.

2 Add to the grill of the air fryer at 350 degrees. Let it grill for a bit.

3 After 20 minutes, take the chicken off and let it cool down before serving.

Nutrition: Calories 375 Fat 18g Carbs 6g Protein 35g

Polish Sausage and Sourdough Kabobs

Basic Recipe

Preparation Time: 5 minutes

Cooking Time: 15 minutes

Servings: 4

Ingredients

1 pound smoked Polish beef sausage, sliced

1 tablespoon mustard

1 tablespoon olive oil tablespoons Worcestershire sauce bell peppers, sliced cups sourdough bread, cubed

Salt and ground black pepper, to taste

Directions:

1 Toss the sausage with the mustard, olive, and Worcestershire sauce. Thread sausage, peppers, and bread onto skewers.

2 Sprinkle with salt and black pepper.

3 Cook in the preheated Air Fryer at 360 degrees F for 11 minutes Brush the skewers with the reserved marinade. Bon appétit!

Nutrition: Calories 284 Fat 13.8g Carbs 16.5g Protein 23.1g

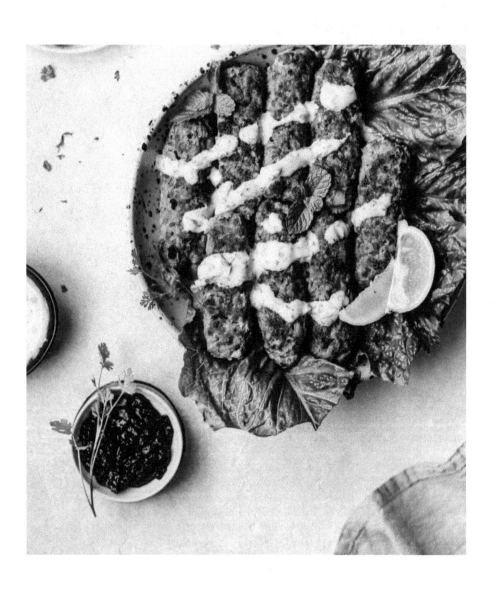

Ranch Meatloaf with Peppers

Basic Recipe

Preparation Time: 5 minutes

Cooking Time: 30 minutes

Servings: 5

Ingredients

1 pound beef, ground

1/2 pound veal, ground

1 egg tablespoons vegetable juice 1 cup crackers, crushed bell peppers, chopped 1 onion, chopped garlic cloves, minced tablespoons tomato paste tablespoons soy sauce

1 (1-ounce) package ranch dressing mix

Sea salt, to taste

1/2 teaspoon ground black pepper, to taste ounces tomato paste

1 tablespoon Dijon mustard

Directions:

1 Start by preheating your Air Fryer to 330 degrees F.

2 In a mixing bowl, thoroughly combine the ground beef, veal, egg, vegetable juice, crackers, bell peppers, onion, garlic, tomato paste, and soy sauce, ranch dressing mix, salt, and ground black pepper. Mix until everything is well incorporated and press into a lightly greased meatloaf pan.

3 Cook approximately 25 minutes in the preheated Air Fryer. Whisk the tomato paste with the mustard and spread the topping over the top of your meatloaf.

4 Continue to cook 2 minutes more. Let it stand on a cooling rack for 6 minutes before slicing and serving. Enjoy!

Nutrition: Calories 411 Fat 31.4g Carbs 10g Protein 28.2g

Indian Beef Samosas

Basic Recipe

Preparation Time: 5 minutes

Cooking Time: 30 minutes

Servings: 8

Ingredients

1 tablespoon sesame oil tablespoons shallots, minced cloves garlic, minced tablespoons green chili peppers, chopped

1/2 pound ground chuck ounces bacon, chopped

Salt and ground black pepper, to taste

1 teaspoon cumin powder

1 teaspoon turmeric

1 teaspoon coriander

1 cup frozen peas, thawed

1 (16-ounce) of phyllo dough

1 egg, beaten with 2 tablespoons of water (egg wash)

Directions:

1 Heat the oil in a saucepan over medium-high heat. Once hot, sauté the shallots, garlic, and chili peppers until tender, about 3 minutes

2 Then, add the beef and bacon; continue to sauté an additional 4 minutes, crumbling with a fork. Season it with salt, pepper, cumin powder, turmeric, and coriander. Stir in peas.

3 Then, preheat your Air Fryer to 330 degrees F. Brush the Air Fryer basket with cooking oil.

4 Place 1 to 2 tablespoons of the mixture onto each phyllo sheet. Fold the sheets into triangles, pressing the edges. Brush the tops with egg wash.

5 Bake it for 7 to 8 minutes, working with batches. Serve with Indian tomato sauce if desired. Enjoy! Nutrition: Calories 266 Fat 13g Carbs 24.5g Protein 12.2g

Yummy Mexican Chicken

Basic Recipe

Preparation Time: 10 minutes

Cooking Time: 15 minutes

Servings: 6

Ingredients

lbs. chicken breasts   tsp cumin   tsp garlic powder   oz. jalapenos, diced   oz. tomatoes, diced

1/2 cup green bell pepper

1/2 cup red bell pepper

1 onion, diced

1 fresh lime juice

2/3 cup chicken broth

1/2 tsp. chili powder

1 tbsp. olive oil

1/4 tsp. salt

Directions:

1. Add oil into the inner pot of air fryer duo crisp and set pot on sauté mode.

2. Add onion, bell peppers and salt and sauté for 3 minutes.

3. Add remaining ingredients and stir well.

4. Seal the pot with pressure cooking lid and cook on high pressure for 12 minutes.

5. Release pressure using a quick release once done. Remove lid.

6. Remove chicken from pot and shred using a fork.

7. Return shredded chicken to the pot and stir well.

8. Serve and enjoy.

Nutrition: Calories 347 Fat 14.2 g Carbs 7.8 g Protein 45.7 g

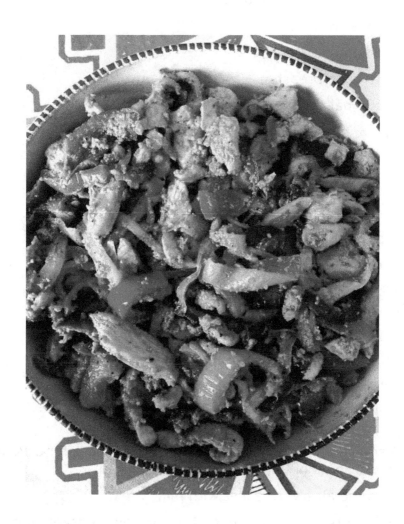

Balsamic Chicken

Basic Recipe

Preparation Time: 10 minutes

Cooking Time: 17 minutes

Servings: 6

Ingredients

lbs. chicken breasts

1/3 cup balsamic vinegar

1 onion, chopped

1/2 cup chicken broth

1 tbsp.Dijon mustard

1/2 tsp. dried thyme

1 tsp. garlic, chopped

Directions:

1 Mix together Dijon, chicken broth, and vinegar and pour into the inner pot of air fryer duo crisp.

2 Add chicken, thyme, garlic, and onion and stir well.

3 Seal the pot with pressure cooking lid and cook on high pressure for 12 minutes.

4 Release pressure using a quick release once done. Remove lid.

5 Remove chicken from pot and shred using a fork. Pour the leftover liquid of pot over shredded chicken.

6 Line the air fryer basket with foil.

7 Add shredded chicken to the air fryer basket and place basket in the pot.

8 Seal the pot with air fryer lid and select broil mode and cook for 5 minutes.

9 Serve and enjoy.

Italian Chicken Wings

Basic Recipe

Preparation Time: 10 minutes

Cooking Time: 15 minutes

Servings: 4 Ingredients

chicken wings

1 tbsp. chicken seasoning tbsp olive oil 1 tbsp. garlic powder

1 tbsp basil 1/2 tbsp. oregano tbsp tarragon

Pepper

Salt

Directions:

1 Add all ingredients into the mixing bowl and toss well.

2 Pour 1 cup water into the inner pot of air fryer duo crisp then place steamer rack in the pot.

3 Arrange chicken wings on top of the steamer rack.

4 Seal the pot with pressure cooking lid and cook on high pressure for 10 minutes.

5 Release pressure using a quick release once done. Remove lid.

6 Remove chicken wings from the pot. Dump leftover liquid from the pot.

7 Add chicken wings into the air fryer basket then place a basket in the pot.

8 Seal the pot with air fryer lid and select broil mode and cook for 5 minutes.

9 Serve and enjoy.

Nutrition: Calories 588 Fat 29.6 g Carbs 2.6 g Protein 74.6 g

Yummy Hawaiian Chicken

Basic Recipe

Preparation Time: 10 minutes

Cooking Time: 12 minutes

Servings: 6

Ingredients

lbs. chicken breasts, skinless, boneless, and cut into chunks tbsp cornstarch 1 cup chicken broth oz. can pineapple tidbits 1 tbsp. garlic, crushed tbsp brown sugar tbsp soy sauce

1/2 tsp. ground ginger

1/2 tsp. salt

Directions:

1 Add all ingredients except cornstarch into the inner pot of air fryer duo crisp and stir well.

2 Seal the pot with pressure cooking lid and cook on high pressure for 10 minutes.

3 Release pressure using a quick release once done. Remove lid. In a small bowl, whisk together 1/4 cup water and cornstarch and pour into the pot.

4 Set pot on sauté mode. Cook chicken on sauce mode until sauce thickens.

5 Serve over rice and enjoy.

Nutrition: Calories 377 Fat 11.5 g Carbs 18.7 g Protein 46 g

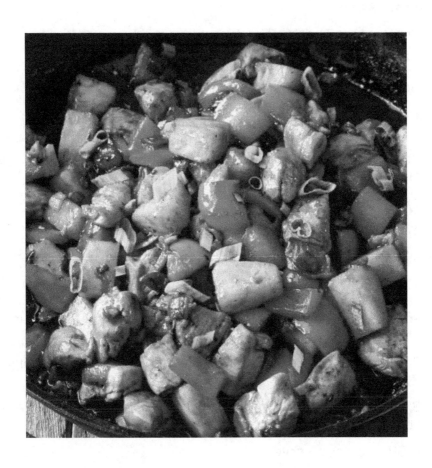

Honey Cashew Butter Chicken

Basic Recipe

Preparation Time: 10 minutes

Cooking Time: 7 minutes

Servings: 3

Ingredients

1 lb. chicken breast, cut into chunks tbsp rice vinegar tbsp honey tbsp coconut aminos 1/4 cup cashew butter garlic cloves, minced

1/4 cup chicken broth

1/2 tbsp. sriracha

Directions:

1 Add chicken into the inner pot of air fryer duo crisp. In a small bowl, mix together cashew butter, garlic, broth, sriracha, vinegar, honey, and coconut aminos and pour over chicken.

2 Seal the pot with pressure cooking lid and cook on high for 7 minutes.

3 Release pressure using a quick release once done. Remove lid.

4 Stir well and serve.

Nutrition: Calories 366 Fat 2.1 g Carbs 20.7 g Protein 36.4 g

Sweet & Tangy Tamarind Chicken

Basic Recipe

Preparation Time: 10 minutes

Cooking Time: 15 minutes

Servings: 4

Ingredients

lbs. chicken breasts, skinless, boneless, and cut into pieces

1 tbsp. ketchup   1 tbsp. vinegar   tbsp ginger, grated   1 garlic clove, minced   tbsp olive oil

1 tbsp. arrowroot powder   1/2 cup tamarind paste

tbsp brown sugar

1 tsp. salt

Directions:

1 Add oil into the inner pot of air fryer duo crisp and set the pot on sauté mode.

2 Add ginger and garlic and sauté for 30 seconds.

3 Add chicken and sauté for 3-4 minutes.

4 In a small bowl, mix together the tamarind paste, brown sugar, ketchup, vinegar, and salt and pour over chicken and stir well.

5 Seal the pot with pressure cooking lid and cook on high for 8 minutes.

6 Release pressure using a quick release once done. Remove lid.

7 In a small bowl, whisk arrowroot powder with 2 tbsp water and pour it into the pot.

8 Set pot on sauté mode and cook chicken for 1-2 minutes.

9 Serve and enjoy.

Nutrition: Calories 598 Fat 27.6 g Carbs 18.9 g Protein 66.4 g

Korean Chicken Wings

Basic Recipe

Preparation Time: 5 minutes

Cooking Time: 10 minutes

Servings: 8 Ingredients Wings:

1 tsp. Pepper

1 tsp. Salt

pounds chicken wings Sauce packets splenda 1 tbsp. Minced garlic

1 tbsp. Minced ginger

1 tbsp. Sesame oil

1 tsp. Agave nectar 1 tbsp. Mayo tbsp. Gochujang

Finishing:

¼ c. Chopped green onions tsp. Sesame seeds

Directions:

1 Ensure instant crisp air fryer is preheated to 400 degrees.

2 Line a small pan with foil and place a rack onto the pan, then place into instant crisp air fryer.

3 Season the wings with pepper and salt and place onto the rack.

4 Lock the air fryer lid. Set temperature to 160°f, and set time to 20 minutes and air fry 20 minutes, turning at 10 minutes.

5 As chicken air fries, mix together all the sauce components.

6 Once a thermometer says that the chicken has reached 160 degrees, take out wings and place into a bowl.

7 Pour half of the sauce mixture over wings, tossing well to coat.

8 Put coated wings back into instant crisp air fryer for 5 minutes or till they reach 165 degrees.

9 Remove and sprinkle with green onions and sesame seeds. Dip into extra sauce.

Nutrition: Calories 356 Fat26g Carbs 21g Protein 23g

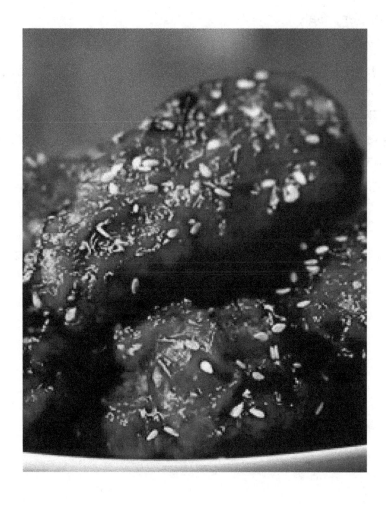

Paprika Chicken

Intermediate Recipe

Preparation Time: 10 minutes

Cooking Time: 30 minutes

Servings: 4 Ingredients

chicken breasts, skinless and boneless, cut into chunks tsp. garlic, minced   tbsp smoked paprika   tbsp olive oil   tbsp lemon juice

Pepper   Salt

Directions:

1 In a small bowl, mix together garlic, lemon juice, paprika, oil, pepper, and salt.

2 Rub chicken with garlic mixture.

3 Add chicken into the air fryer air fryer basket and place basket in the pot.

4 Seal the pot with air fryer lid and select bake mode and cook at 350 f for 30 minutes.

5 Serve and enjoy.

Nutrition: Calories 381 Fat 21.8 g Carbs 2.6 g Protein 42.9 g

Garlic Lemon Chicken

Intermediate Recipe

Preparation Time: 10 minutes

Cooking Time: 40 minutes

Servings: 4 Ingredients

lbs. chicken drumsticks   tbsp   butter   tbsp   parsley, chopped   1 fresh lemon juice   garlic cloves, minced   tbsp olive oil

Pepper   Salt

Directions:

1 Add butter, parsley, lemon juice, garlic, oil, pepper, and salt into the mixing bowl and mix well.

2 Add chicken to the bowl and toss until well coated.

3 Transfer chicken into the air fryer air fryer basket and place basket in the pot.

4 Seal the pot with air fryer lid and select bake mode and cook at 400 f for 40 minutes.

5 Serve and enjoy.

Nutrition: Calories 560 Fat 31.6 g Carbs 2.9 g Protein 63.1 g

Flavorful Herb Chicken

Intermediate Recipe

Preparation Time: 10 minutes

Cooking Time: 4 hours

Servings: 6

Ingredients

chicken breasts, skinless and boneless

1 onion, sliced   oz. can tomato, diced   1 tsp. dried basil

1 tsp. dried rosemary

1 tbsp. olive oil

1/2 cup balsamic vinegar

1/2 tsp. thyme   1 tsp. dried oregano   garlic cloves

Pepper   Salt

Directions:

1 Add all ingredients into the inner pot of air fryer duo crisp and stir well.

2 Seal the pot with pressure cooking lid and select slow cook mode and cook on high for 4 hours.

3 Stir well and serve.

Nutrition: Calories 328 Fat 13.3 g Carbs 6.3 g Protein 43.2 g

Chicken and Potatoes

Preparation Time: 1 hour

Cooking Time: 55 minutes

Servings: 2

Ingredients

Pepper and salt

Provencal herbs

Chicken pieces

Potatoes

Olive oil

Directions:

1 Peel the skin from the potatoes and cut into slices. Add some pepper and place into the air fryer.

2 Preheat to 340 degrees. Cover the chicken with the herbs, pepper, salt, and oil and add it in with the potatoes.

3 Cook this until well done. After forty minutes, turn the chicken around and let it cook another 15 minutes before serving.

Nutrition: Calories 200 Carbs 18g Fat 4g Protein 22g

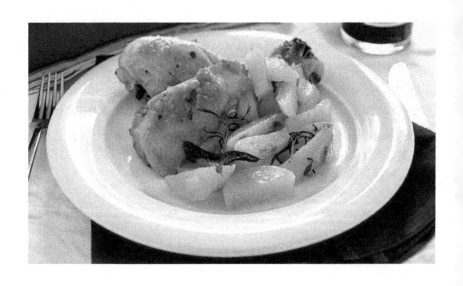

Coconut-Crusted Chicken Tenders

Preparation Time: 15 minutes

Cooking Time: 8 minutes

Servings: 4

Ingredients

Eggs

1 lb. Chicken tenders 1 cup Cornstarch

cups. Sweetened shredded coconut

1 tsp. Cayenne pepper

Directions:

1 Set the Air Fryer temperature at 360° Fahrenheit.

2 Prepare three dishes. In the first one, add the cornstarch and cayenne with any other desired seasonings. In the second bowl, add the eggs. Lastly, add the coconut in the third dish.

3 Dredge the chicken through the cornstarch, egg, and coconut.

4 Lightly spritz the fryer basket with a cooking oil spray as needed.

5 Set the timer for 8 minutes and air-fry until it's golden brown before serving.

Nutrition: Calories: 390 kcal Protein: 32.38 g Fat: 12.14 g Carbohydrates: 34.67 g

Crispy Chicken Sliders

Preparation Time: 10 minutes

Cooking Time: 8 minutes

Servings: 6

Ingredients

1 pkg. Tyson Crispy Chicken Strips

1 pkg. Sweet Hawaiian Rolls

Optional Ingredients

Spinach leaves

Tomatoes

Honey mustard

Directions:

1 Place the six chicken strips in the Air Fryer basket with a coating of olive oil spray. Cook at 390º Fahrenheit for 8 minutes.

2 Slice the rolls in half and top them with honey mustard, spinach, and tomatoes or other toppings of your choice.

3 Slice the chicken strips into chunks and place them on the rolls.

Nutrition: Calories: 53 kcal Protein: 3.9 g Fat: 3.27 g Carbohydrates: 1.87 g

Garlic Herb Turkey Breast

Preparation Time: 1 hour

Cooking Time: 40 minutes

Servings: 6

Ingredients

lb. Turkey breast tbsp. Melted butter cloves Garlic 1 tsp. Thyme

1 tsp. Rosemary

Directions:

1 Warm the Air Fryer to reach 375° Fahrenheit.

2 Pat the turkey breast dry. Mince the garlic and chop the rosemary and thyme.

3 Melt the butter and mix with the garlic, thyme, and rosemary in a small mixing bowl. Brush the butter over turkey breast.

4 Place in the Air Fryer basket, skin side up, and cook for 40 minutes or until internal temperature reaches 160° Fahrenheit, flipping halfway through.

5 Wait for five minutes before slicing.

Nutrition: Calories: 321 kcal Protein: 34.35 g Fat: 19.32 g Carbohydrates: 0.56 g

Honey-Lime Chicken Wings

Preparation Time: 20 minutes

Cooking Time: 30 minutes

Servings: 4

Ingredients

lb. Chicken wings tbsp. Lime juice .25 cup Honey

1 tbsp. Lime zest

1 pressed Garlic clove

Directions:

1 Warm the Air Fryer at 360° Fahrenheit.

2 Whisk the garlic, honey, and lime juice and zest. Toss in the wings and cover with the mixture.

3 Prepare the wings in batches. Cook for 25-30 minutes until they're crispy. Shake the basket at 8-minute intervals.

4 Serve and garnish as desired.

Nutrition: Calories: 375 kcal Protein: 51.59 g Fat: 9.56 g Carbohydrates: 18.67 g

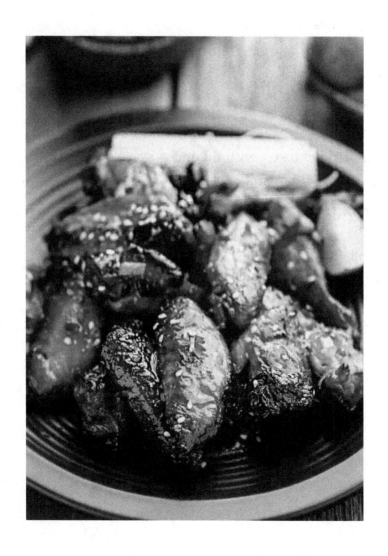

Rotisserie-Style, Whole Chicken

Preparation Time: 50 minutes

Cooking Time: 30 minutes

Servings: 4

Ingredients

tsp. Olive oil, as needed 6-7 lb. Whole chicken

1 tbsp. Seasoned salt

Directions:

1 Set the Air Fryer at 350° Fahrenheit.

2 Coat the chicken with oil and a sprinkle of salt.

3 Arrange the chicken in the Air Fryer – skin-side down.

4 Cook for 30 minutes. Flip the chicken over and air-fry for another 30 minutes.

5 Wait for ten minutes before slicing

6 Note: This recipe is for chickens under 6 lb. for a 3.7-quart Air Fryer.

Nutrition: Calories: 859 kcal Protein: 151.45 g Fat: 23.67 g Carbohydrates: 0 g

Cheeseburger 'Mini' Sliders

Preparation Time: 15 minutes

Cooking Time: 10 minutes

Servings: 1

Ingredients

　　slices Cheddar cheese

1 lb. Ground beef

Freshly cracked black pepper and salt (as desired)

Dinner rolls

Directions:

1 Warm the Air Fryer ahead of fry time to 390º Fahrenheit.

2 Shape six (2.5-oz.) patties and dust with the pepper and salt

3 Arrange the burgers in the fryer basket and cook for ten minutes.

4 Take them out of the cooker and add the cheese.

5 Return them to the basket for another minute until the cheese melts.

Nutrition: Calories: 382 kcal Protein: 35.62 g Fat: 16.77 g Carbohydrates: 20.38 g

Quick and Easy Rib Eye Steak

Preparation Time: 40 minutes

Cooking Time: 35 minutes

Servings: 2

Ingredients

lb. Unchilled steak

1 tbsp. Olive oil

Steak Rub: Salt and pepper mix (desired)

Baking pan also needed to fit into the basket

Directions:

1 Press the "M" button for the French Fries icon. Adjust the time to four minutes at 400° Fahrenheit.

2 Rub the steak with the oil and seasonings. Arrange the steak in the basket and air-fry for 14 minutes. (Flip it over after seven minutes.)

3 Place the rib eye on a platter, and let it rest for ten minutes.

4 Slice it and garnish the way you like it.

Nutrition: Calories: 1017 kcal Protein: 129.44 g Fat: 55.78 g Carbohydrates: 0 g

Roast Beef

Preparation Time: 1 hour

Cooking Time: 55 minutes

Servings: 6

Ingredients

.5 tsp. Garlic powder

.5 tsp. Oregano

1 tsp. Dried thyme 1 tbsp. Olive oil lb. Round roast

Directions:

1 Heat the Air Fryer at 330º Fahrenheit.

2 Combine the spices. Brush the oil over the beef, and rub it using the spice mixture.

3 Add to a baking dish and arrange it in the Air Fryer basket for 30 minutes. Turn it over and continue cooking 25 more minutes.

4 Wait for a few minutes before slicing.

5 Serve on your choice of bread or plain with a delicious side dish.

Nutrition: Calories: 287 kcal Protein: 45.97 g Fat: 10.01 g Carbohydrates: 0.28 g

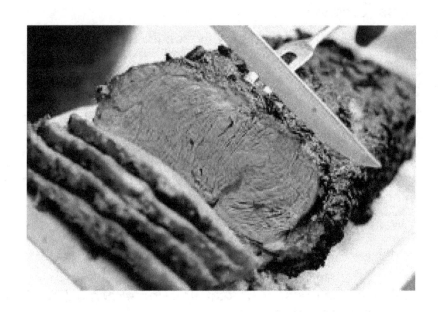

Sweet and Spicy Montreal Steak

Preparation Time: 30 minutes

Cooking Time: 6 minutes

Servings: 2

Ingredients

boneless Sirloin steaks 1 tbsp. Brown sugar

1 tbsp. Montreal steak seasoning

1 tsp. Crushed red pepper

1 tbsp. Olive oil

Directions:

1 Set the temperature of the Air Fryer at 390º Fahrenheit.

2 Prepare the steaks with oil. Rub them with the desired seasonings.

3 Arrange the steaks in the basket and set the timer for three minutes.

4 Flip the steak over and air-fry for another three minutes.

5 Cool and slice it into strips before serving.

Nutrition: Calories: 1253 kcal Protein: 126.25 g Fat: 75.9 g Carbohydrates: 6.58 g

Bacon-Wrapped Pork Tenderloin

Preparation Time: 1 hour Cooking Time:

Servings: 4 to 6

Ingredients

1 lb. Pork tenderloin

1-2 tbsp. Dijon mustard

3-4 strips Bacon

Directions:

1 Set the Air Fryer temperature at 360º Fahrenheit.

2 Coat the tenderloin with the mustard and wrap with the bacon.

3 Air-fry them for 15 minutes. Flip and cook 10 to 15 more minutes.

4 Serve with your favorite sides.

Nutrition: Calories: 133 kcal Protein: 21.31 g Fat: 4.65 g Carbohydrates: 0.41 g

Spicy Green Crusted Chicken

Preparation Time: 10 minutes

Cooking Time: 40 minutes

Servings: 4

Ingredients

whole eggs, beaten teaspoons parsley teaspoons thyme teaspoons paprika ¾ pound chicken pieces Salt and pepper, to taste teaspoons oregano

Directions:

1 Preheat your air fryer to 360 degrees F.

2 Grease the air fryer cooking basket.

3 Crack eggs in a bowl and whisk well, take another bowl and mix all of the ingredients except chicken pieces.

4 Dip chicken in eggs and then into the dry mixture.

5 Transfer half of the chicken pieces to your air fryer and cook for 20 minutes.

6 Keep repeating until all ingredients are used up.

7 Enjoy!

Nutrition: Calories: 393 Total Fat: 22g Total Carbs: 7g Fiber: 1g Net Carbs: 4g Protein: 39g

Cheesy Chicken Drumsticks

Preparation Time: 18 minutes

Cooking Time: 15 minutes

Servings: 2

Ingredients

1-pound small chicken drumsticks, bone-in tablespoons almond flour 1 cup mixed cheese, grated

1 teaspoon dried rosemary

1 teaspoon dried oregano

½ teaspoon chili flakes

½ teaspoon salt

½ teaspoon pepper

Chopped green onion for garnish

Directions:

1 Rinse drumsticks thoroughly and pat them dry.

2 Take a medium-sized bowl and add flour, mixed cheese, herbs, chili flakes, salt, and pepper.

3 Dip drumsticks in the mixture and turn them well, keep in the freezer for 5 minutes.

4 Spray air fryer cooking basket with cooking spray and preheat your fryer to 370 degrees F.

5 Transfer drumsticks to your fryer and cook for 15 minutes, making sure to shake the basket halfway through.

6 Transfer to a serving plate, and enjoy with your garnish!

Nutrition: Calories: 226 Total Fat: 10g Total Carbs: 4g Fiber: 1g Net Carbs: 2g Protein: 16g

Bratwurst and Veggies

Preparation Time: 10 minutes

Cooking Time: 20 minutes

Servings: 2

Ingredients

1 pkg. Bratwurst

1 each Red and green bell pepper .25 cup Onion - red or purple tbsp. Gluten-free Cajun seasoning

Directions:

1 Warm the unit to reach 390° Fahrenheit.

2 Line the Air Fryer with foil, if preferred.

3 Slice and add in the vegetables.

4 Slice the bratwurst into about 0.5-inch size rounds, and place on top of the veggies.

5 Evenly sprinkle the seasoning on top.

6 Air-fry for 10 minutes. Carefully open and stir or mix.

7 Air-fry for another 10 minutes before serving.

Nutrition: Calories: 84 kcal Protein: 1.57 g Fat: 0.06 g Carbohydrates: 15.89 g

CPSIA information can be obtained
at www.ICGtesting.com
Printed in the USA
BVHW090228280421
605947BV00002B/567